BOOKENDING YOUR DAY

THE LIGHTHOUSE EFFECT

Self-Care 30-day Challenge

by

Faith Burrington Jones

ISBN: 979-8-9904262-0-7

Printed in the USA

Cover & Interior Images Canva Pro | Edit & Design Linda Black

THE LIGHTHOUSE EFFECT™

FAITH BURRINGTON JONES

THE LIGHTHOUSE EFFECT™

The Lighthouse Effect is the Skillful Recovery Program I developed over many years, originally as a group-therapy process to guide people through recovery from addiction, co-occurring mental health challenges, codependency, and early trauma. It evolved into a training program to support second stage recovery, recovery coaches, and addiction counselors, as presented in *The Lighthouse Effect Training Guide*.

The training program focuses on second stage recovery, which is where you deepen your healing by exploring the underlying mental and emotional barriers to health and wellbeing. The training guide walks you through the program's five modules: Mindful Recovery, Tolerance Building, Emotional Balancing, Effective Interpersonal Communication, and the Integration module, where you incorporate all that you've learned and formulate your custom daily practice ~ Bookending Your Day.

The Lighthouse Effect companion book is a collection of authentic and inspirational recovery stories from some of the people who participated in and graduated from the program. It also includes a deeper exploration of recovery, healing concepts, and inspirational quotes, and I share my own process of how I came to this work.

Video recordings of all five modules of The Lighthouse Effect Skillful Recovery Program are available on my website (www.innerfaiththerapy.com) along with guided meditations, events calendar, my "Innerfaith Therapy" services, and more.

Faith Burrington Jones

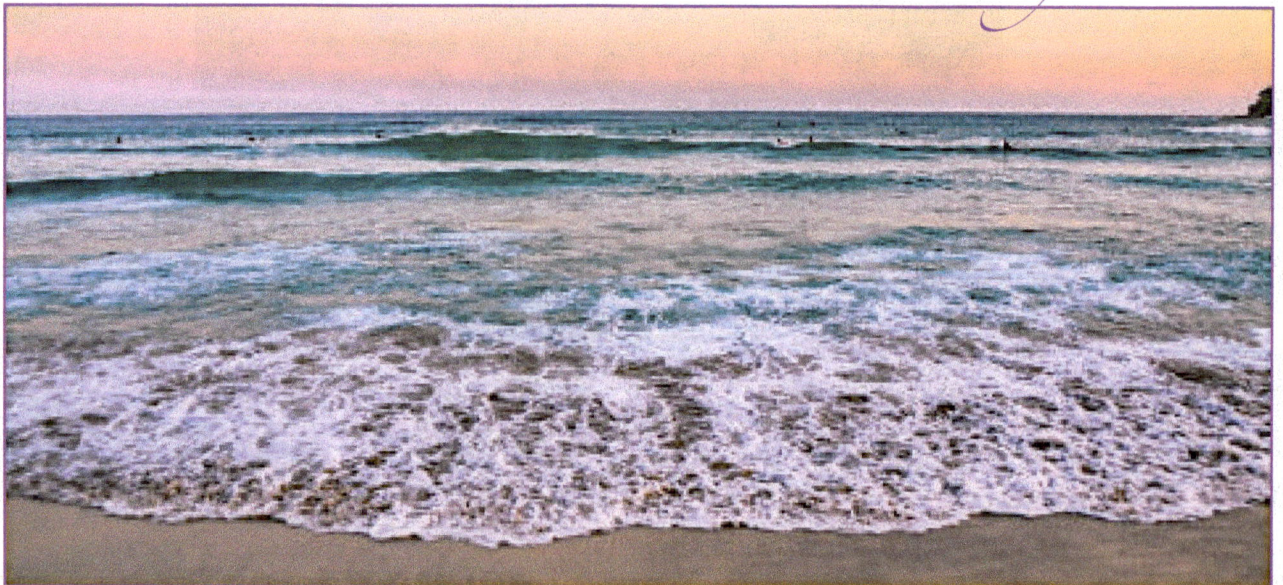

BOOKENDING YOUR DAY

Do you care for yourself as well as you care for others? Through decades of practicing and reflecting on the benefits of doing inner work and working with others in trauma and addiction, I have noticed that the common denominator seems to be an almost instinctual inability to self-love and to fully get to know our selves. (Underscores the ancient philosophical maxim, *know thyself*!) What does it look like to come to know yourself and your true worth? What does it mean to *love* yourself?

Bookending Your Day (B.E.D.) is an exercise implemented in my Skillful Recovery Program that addresses those questions. It can be used by anyone as a daily practice because we are all recovering from something (childhood programming, trauma, loss of a loved one, mental or physical health challenges, life transitions, life situations) or are simply wanting to improve the quality of care we give to ourselves. This thirty- day challenge is an invitation to live your life with purpose and intention. Putting energy into *you* might be challenging, but it is also quite simple. It is simply about you giving yourself what you want or need, instead of waiting for someone or something outside of you to do it for you.

Mind/Body/Spirit ~ Thoughts/Words/Deeds

You are the one you have been waiting for. This B.E.D. practice is about beginning and ending your day in ways that work for you, so you can radiate your unique expression of Self. Rather than focusing on and reacting to what's coming at you from the horizontal plane, choose to center yourself vertically-between earth and sky-to come into your essential self, or soul self. Turn inward to deeply listen and connect with your Higher Power. Mind/body/ spirit integration is essential to self-care. Think of the mind, body, and spirit as your "books" (essentially, a trilogy) and this bookending practice as how you might "hold" or align them. Mind, as in how you judge and think about yourself (self-talk). Body, how you take care of your body (food, exercise, boundaries, environment). Spirit, how you connect with non-physical reality, with your soul (what nourishes you on a deep emotional level, where you are aligned with the frequency of Love). The idea is to "make it simple" so you can "make it happen." You might ask, make what happen?

Whatever you want or need *today* to support your health and wellbeing. Because today is the only day you can *actually* experience. What turns you (your mind/body/spirit) on or inspires you? How do you decompress or reduce stress? Spending time with family, friends, or an animal, or being in nature? This is about you creating your own instruction manual to work and function your best, to be your best self, to integrate mind/body/spirit. Let's begin!

MORNING BOOKEND

Mind will follow Body: You may notice that in the morning ritual there is a different order for setting yourself up for alignment of mind/body/spirit. With the thinking that it can take the mind a little time to wake up and that "mind will follow body," the morning ritual looks to the body first, so body/mind/spirit. You can determine what works best for you as you customize your self-care practice. The prompts in the daily worksheets are like buoys in a harbor that can help you navigate and inspire you to create your own personalized prompts.

I am Light ~ I am Love ~ I am Truth ~ I am

What seems to work for most is to begin the day with a "best way to be" mindset. Ask yourself: *What will work best for me today*? Set an intention for the day that considers how you will think and act toward yourself and others, how you will move and nourish your body, and how you will connect with Spirit or Higher Self.

This is my opportunity to take myself through the day with purpose and with intention. This is truly the one and only day I have. Yesterday is gone and tomorrow isn't here yet – and once it arrives, "tomorrow" changes to "today." Essentially all I ever have is today!

Bookend your day with your custom morning ritual. Make it simple yet powerful!

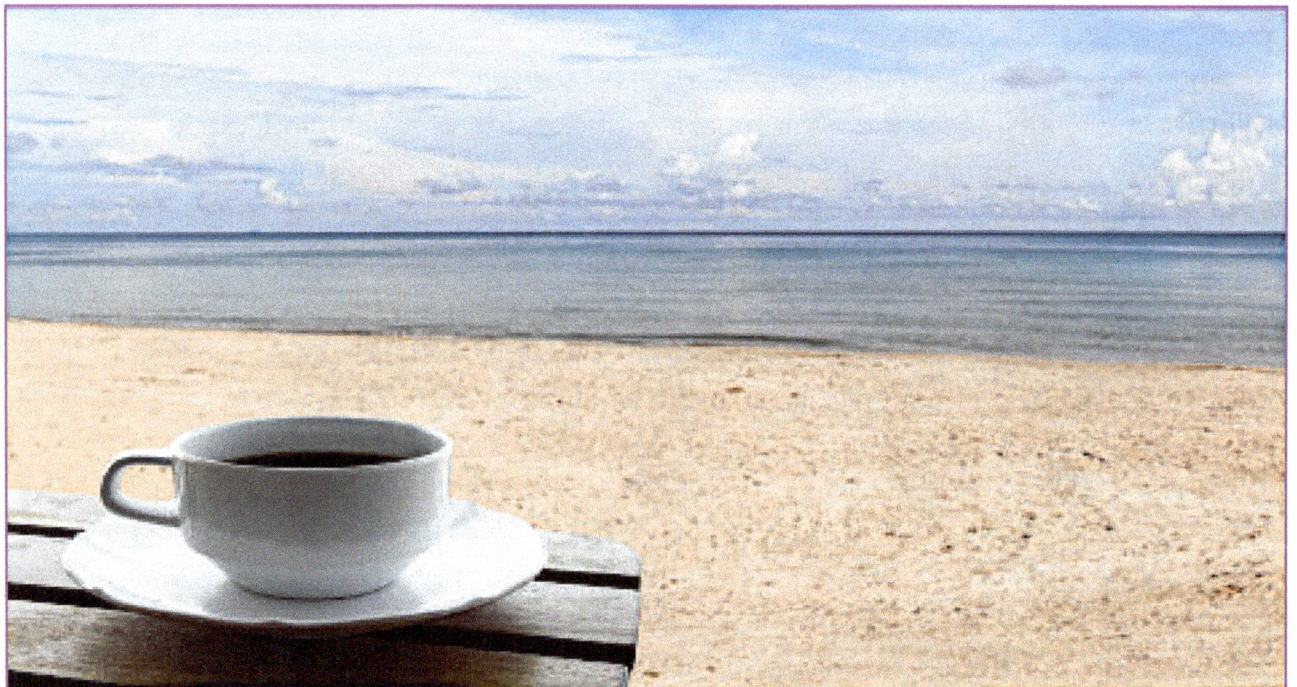

MORNING RITUAL

✦

BODY

Nourish your Body: You might start with some slow, deep breaths and gentle stretching in bed. Move slowly, like a cat getting up from a nap. Then think about how you will move, nurture, and fuel your body throughout the day. What exercises or activities work best for you? Taking a walk, doing yoga, qigong? What will you eat that is nutritious and healing? (Or would it be healing for you to do intermittent fasting to rest your digestive system?)

MIND

Be mindful with your "Self-Talk:" Mindful self-talking is about talking to yourself in a kind, supportive way. If you catch yourself not being kind, reframe your thoughts, comments, or judgments to make them more forgiving and supportive.

I will start off my day being kind and accepting toward myself. I will speak to myself with utmost respect and kindness. Even if I didn't sleep well last night, I will take extra good care of myself and make it a good day, as best I can.

SPIRIT

Create a mantra: Say it to yourself upon rising, and throughout the day. It might be a "mind stretch" and something to aspire to, like the "I am Light" mantra on the previous page. Or it could be something that will remind you to be patient, kind, and caring toward yourself. If you choose to use the words of inspiration provided on each day's morning ritual, I encourage you to still write them down to help ground the idea and manifest it in your being.

I am worthy of love and I am willing to seek relationships that encourage mutual growth and wellbeing. Only I can choose to gift myself with people, places, and practices that support me and mirror back my unique spirit.

Remind yourself you are a spiritual being having a human experience. Whenever you get a break during the day, take a moment to let go of negative narratives playing in your mind. Take a deep breath, look in the mirror, and assure yourself, *"I've got this!"*

EVENING BOOKEND

Before we ease into the Evening Bookend, let's look at one of the ways you can support yourself in your B.E.D. journey. I highly recommend that you share your process with an accountability partner or guide, someone of your careful choosing who you trust would be respectful and provide gentle encouragement, just as you are attempting to do in "practicing" to be with yourself in this new way.

If they experience you reverting to old, judgmental, or self-deprecating patterns, have them remind you to be kind and forgiving to your Self. For example, *I wonder if there is another way you could share this with me*? Or, *could you please say that again with a softer tone or in a different way, without negative language*?

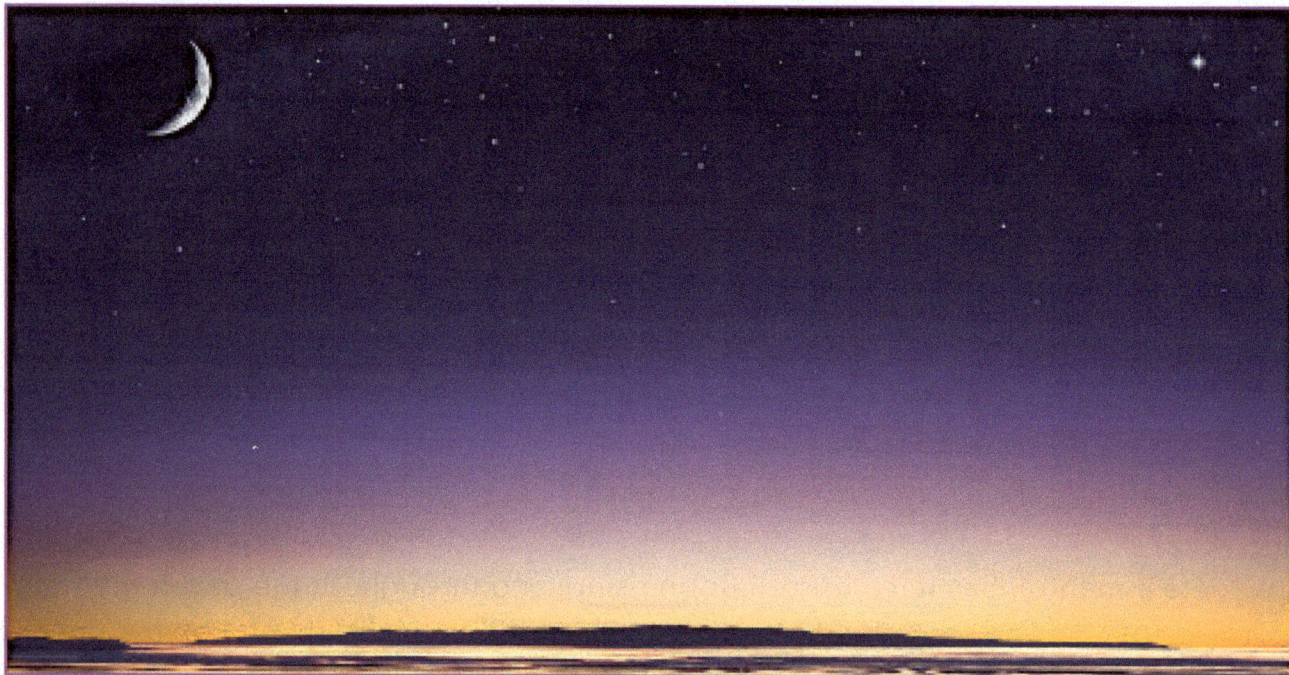

The evening or bedtime ritual is essential to improving the quality of your sleep (and your energy level when you awaken). Remember, you only get one day at a time, so why not put every effort into readying yourself for restful sleep?

What will you do tonight to best prepare your Self for your new "today?" You could start by moving your devices to another room, as their Electromagnetic Field emissions can cause restlessness and insomnia. Think of other ways to slowly bring your day to a close. What works for you? Listening to comforting meditations, or reading? (If you are going to read before bed, choose something that will help you feel safe and comforted, perhaps a book or poetry or spiritual stories.)

EVENING RITUAL

✦

MIND

Slow your mind down: Read, meditate, or listen to meditations or soft music. Any of these can work to "quiet the mind." Evenings are also a good time to journal and reflect on your day. Let go of any conflicts and set aside unfinished projects; you can revisit them on the next "today."

BODY

Reassure yourself that we all are just doing our best as spiritual beings in this human experience. That includes you! You have earned a restful sleep. Choose to be kind and gentle with your Self, and give yourself what you need to make it happen.

Slow your body down: Try to not watch TV or scroll social media just prior to sleep. It can be overstimulating because the blue light (photo-toxicity) from your device penetrates your retinas, and the downloads of information tax the mind and body.

Take an evening walk or do some gentle stretches. Use aromatherapy: Light a candle infused with essence of lavender or take a hot bath with lavender and Epson salts. Have a cup of chamomile tea or another calming herbal tea to help sedate the body, calm the senses, and prepare you for restful sleep.

SPIRIT

Connect with your Soul Self: Recite your mantra from the morning ritual or make a new one to end your day.

Feel *held* in your bed by making it cozy and warm, or cool and refreshing, whatever your preference. What can you do to achieve that? Tuck a hot-water bottle by your feet? Put fresh sheets on your bed?

Feeling safe and held in your bed will help you fall into the arms of sleep. Call upon your Soul Self (Higher Power/God/Source Energy) to support you in letting go of the waking world and help lead you into a rejuvenating rest.

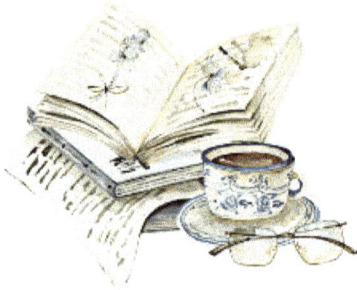

DAY ONE

✦

MORNING RITUAL

BODY: I will first take slow, deep breaths and do gentle stretches in bed. What other exercise or activity will I do? What nourishing foods will I provide myself with today?

_____
_____
_____
_____
_____
_____
_____
_____

Self-care is not selfishness ~ it is soulfullness

MIND: How will I choose to talk to myself and about myself today, even if something is off or not working? (I will practice self-acceptance and self-forgiveness, and be kind.)

_____
_____
_____
_____
_____
_____
_____
_____

SPIRIT: I will be open to receiving signs from Spirit today. What inspirational affirmation, prayer, or mantra will guide me through my day?

_____
_____
_____
_____
_____
_____
_____
_____

DAY ONE

✦

EVENING RITUAL

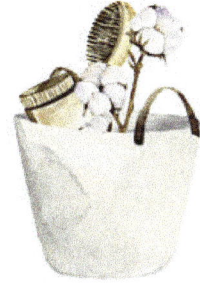

MIND: How did I do today, with treating myself with kindness? What worked? What felt good? How did I take care of myself?

_____
_____
_____
_____
_____
_____
_____
_____
_____

BODY: How did I or how will I prepare my body for a restful sleep tonight?

_____
_____
_____
_____
_____
_____
_____
_____
_____
_____

SPIRIT: What signs did I receive from Spirit today? What words of affirmation, mantra, or prayer will I say to myself, to quiet my mind and help me ease into a restful sleep?

_____
_____
_____
_____
_____
_____
_____
_____

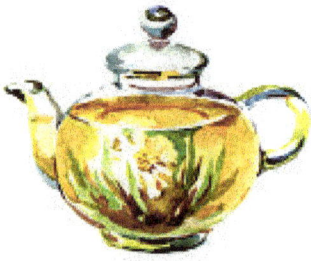

DAY TWO

✦

MORNING RITUAL

BODY: I will first take slow, deep breaths and do gentle stretches in bed. What other exercise or activity will I do? What nourishing foods will I provide myself with today?

_____
_____
_____
_____
_____
_____
_____
_____
_____

I will flow with whatever life brings today

MIND: How will I choose to talk to myself and about myself today, even if something is off or not working? (I will practice self-acceptance and self-forgiveness, and be kind.)

_____
_____
_____
_____
_____
_____
_____
_____
_____

SPIRIT: I will be open to receiving signs from Spirit today. What inspirational affirmation, prayer, or mantra will guide me through my day?

_____
_____
_____
_____
_____
_____
_____
_____
_____

DAY TWO

✦

EVENING RITUAL

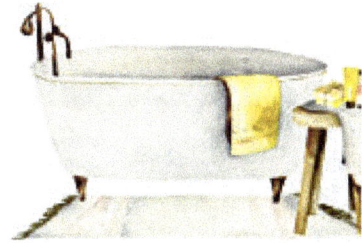

MIND: How did I do today, with treating myself with kindness? What worked? What felt good? How did I take care of myself?

_____
_____
_____
_____
_____
_____
_____
_____
_____

BODY: How did I or how will I prepare my body for a restful sleep tonight?

_____
_____
_____
_____
_____
_____
_____
_____
_____
_____
_____

SPIRIT: What signs did I receive from Spirit today? What words of affirmation, mantra, or prayer will I say to myself, to quiet my mind and help me ease into a restful sleep?

_____
_____
_____
_____
_____
_____
_____
_____

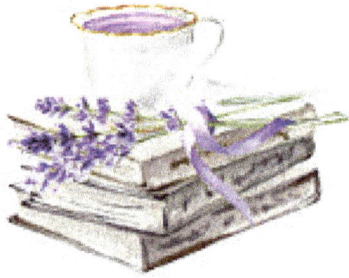

DAY THREE

✦

MORNING RITUAL

BODY: I will first take slow, deep breaths and do gentle stretches in bed. What other exercise or activity will I do? What nourishing foods will I provide myself with today?

_____
_____
_____
_____
_____
_____
_____
_____

I am a spiritual being having a human experience

MIND: How will I choose to talk to myself and about myself today, even if something is off or not working? (I will practice self-acceptance and self-forgiveness, and be kind.)

_____
_____
_____
_____
_____
_____
_____
_____
_____

SPIRIT: I will be open to receiving signs from Spirit today. What inspirational affirmation, prayer, or mantra will guide me through my day?

_____
_____
_____
_____
_____
_____
_____
_____

DAY THREE

✦

EVENING RITUAL

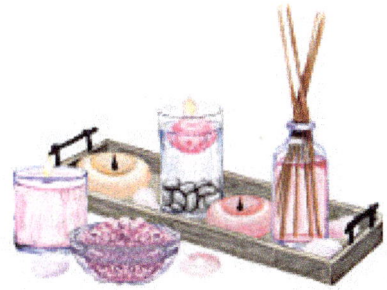

MIND: How did I do today, with treating myself with kindness? What worked? What felt good? How did I take care of myself?

_____
_____
_____
_____
_____
_____
_____
_____
_____
_____

BODY: How did I or how will I prepare my body for a restful sleep tonight?

_____
_____
_____
_____
_____
_____
_____
_____
_____
_____

SPIRIT: What signs did I receive from Spirit today? What words of affirmation, mantra, or prayer will I say to myself, to quiet my mind and help me ease into a restful sleep?

_____
_____
_____
_____
_____
_____
_____
_____
_____
_____

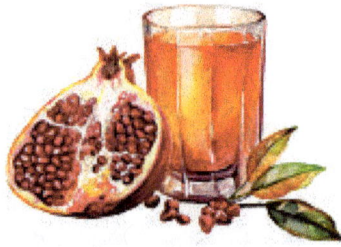

DAY FOUR

✦

MORNING RITUAL

BODY: I will first take slow, deep breaths and do gentle stretches in bed. What other exercise or activity will I do? What nourishing foods will I provide myself with today?

_____
_____
_____
_____
_____
_____
_____
_____
_____

I choose peace over conflict

MIND: How will I choose to talk to myself and about myself today, even if something is off or not working? (I will practice self-acceptance and self-forgiveness, and be kind.)

_____
_____
_____
_____
_____
_____
_____
_____
_____

SPIRIT: I will be open to receiving signs from Spirit today. What inspirational affirmation, prayer, or mantra will guide me through my day?

_____
_____
_____
_____
_____
_____
_____
_____
_____

DAY FOUR

✦

EVENING RITUAL

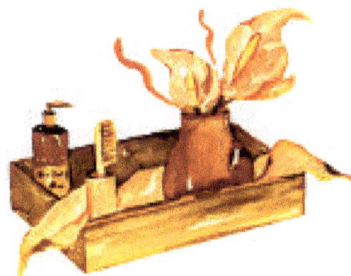

MIND: How did I do today, with treating myself with kindness? What worked? What felt good? How did I take care of myself?

_____
_____
_____
_____
_____
_____
_____
_____
_____
_____

BODY: How did I or how will I prepare my body for a restful sleep tonight?

_____
_____
_____
_____
_____
_____
_____
_____
_____
_____

SPIRIT: What signs did I receive from Spirit today? What words of affirmation, mantra, or prayer will I say to myself, to quiet my mind and help me ease into a restful sleep?

_____
_____
_____
_____
_____
_____
_____
_____
_____
_____

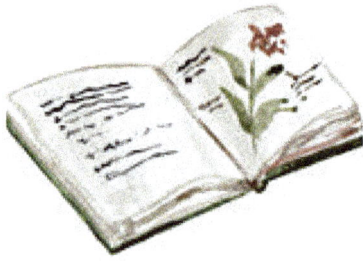

DAY FIVE

✦

MORNING RITUAL

BODY: I will first take slow, deep breaths and do gentle stretches in bed. What other exercise or activity will I do? What nourishing foods will I provide myself with today?

_____
_____
_____
_____
_____
_____
_____
_____

If I am not good to myself,
how can I expect anyone else to be good to me?

– Maya Angelou

MIND: How will I choose to talk to myself and about myself today, even if something is off or not working? (I will practice self-acceptance and self-forgiveness, and be kind.)

_____
_____
_____
_____
_____
_____
_____
_____

SPIRIT: I will be open to receiving signs from Spirit today. What inspirational affirmation, prayer, or mantra will guide me through my day?

_____
_____
_____
_____
_____
_____
_____

DAY FIVE

✦

EVENING RITUAL

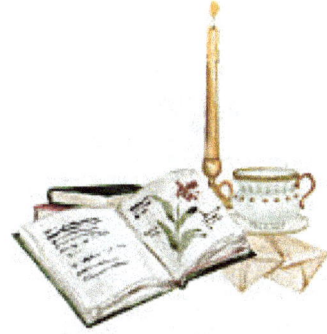

MIND: How did I do today, with treating myself with kindness? What worked? What felt good? How did I take care of myself?

_____
_____
_____
_____
_____
_____
_____
_____
_____

BODY: How did I or how will I prepare my body for a restful sleep tonight?

_____
_____
_____
_____
_____
_____
_____
_____
_____
_____

SPIRIT: What signs did I receive from Spirit today? What words of affirmation, mantra, or prayer will I say to myself, to quiet my mind and help me ease into a restful sleep?

_____
_____
_____
_____
_____
_____
_____
_____
_____

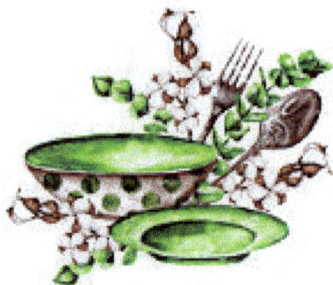

DAY SIX

✦

MORNING RITUAL

BODY: I will first take slow, deep breaths and do gentle stretches in bed. What other exercise or activity will I do? What nourishing foods will I provide myself with today?

_____
_____
_____
_____
_____
_____
_____
_____
_____

I align with my Soul rather than my Ego

MIND: How will I choose to talk to myself and about myself today, even if something is off or not working? (I will practice self-acceptance and self-forgiveness, and be kind.)

_____
_____
_____
_____
_____
_____
_____
_____
_____

SPIRIT: I will be open to receiving signs from Spirit today. What inspirational affirmation, prayer, or mantra will guide me through my day?

_____
_____
_____
_____
_____
_____
_____
_____
_____
_____

DAY SIX

✦

EVENING RITUAL

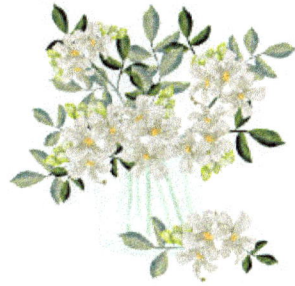

MIND: How did I do today, with treating myself with kindness? What worked? What felt good? How did I take care of myself?

_____
_____
_____
_____
_____
_____
_____
_____
_____

BODY: How did I or how will I prepare my body for a restful sleep tonight?

_____
_____
_____
_____
_____
_____
_____
_____
_____
_____

SPIRIT: What signs did I receive from Spirit today? What words of affirmation, mantra, or prayer will I say to myself, to quiet my mind and help me ease into a restful sleep?

_____
_____
_____
_____
_____
_____
_____
_____
_____

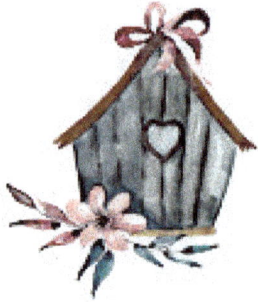

DAY SEVEN

✦

MORNING RITUAL

BODY: I will first take slow, deep breaths and do gentle stretches in bed. What other exercise or activity will I do? What nourishing foods will I provide myself with today?

_____
_____
_____
_____
_____
_____
_____
_____

I will meet myself with understanding and forgiveness

MIND: How will I choose to talk to myself and about myself today, even if something is off or not working? (I will practice self-acceptance and self-forgiveness, and be kind.)

_____
_____
_____
_____
_____
_____
_____
_____
_____

SPIRIT: I will be open to receiving signs from Spirit today. What inspirational affirmation, prayer, or mantra will guide me through my day?

_____
_____
_____
_____
_____
_____
_____
_____

DAY SEVEN

✦

EVENING RITUAL

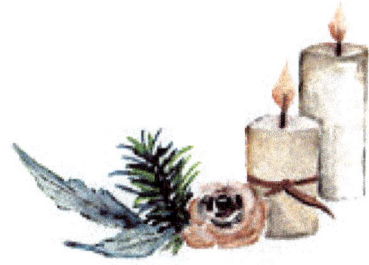

MIND: How did I do today, with treating myself with kindness? What worked? What felt good? How did I take care of myself?

_____
_____
_____
_____
_____
_____
_____
_____
_____
_____

BODY: How did I or how will I prepare my body for a restful sleep tonight?

_____
_____
_____
_____
_____
_____
_____
_____
_____
_____
_____

SPIRIT: What signs did I receive from Spirit today? What words of affirmation, mantra, or prayer will I say to myself, to quiet my mind and help me ease into a restful sleep?

_____
_____
_____
_____
_____
_____
_____
_____
_____
_____

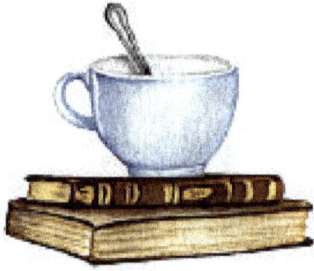

DAY EIGHT

✦

MORNING RITUAL

BODY: I will first take slow, deep breaths and do gentle stretches in bed. What other exercise or activity will I do? What nourishing foods will I provide myself with today?

_____
_____
_____
_____
_____
_____
_____
_____
_____

Love is not a feeling ~ it's a willingness

– David Whyte

MIND: How will I choose to talk to myself and about myself today, even if something is off or not working? (I will practice self-acceptance and self-forgiveness, and be kind.)

_____
_____
_____
_____
_____
_____
_____
_____

SPIRIT: I will be open to receiving signs from Spirit today. What inspirational affirmation, prayer, or mantra will guide me through my day?

_____
_____
_____
_____
_____
_____
_____
_____
_____

DAY EIGHT

✦

EVENING RITUAL

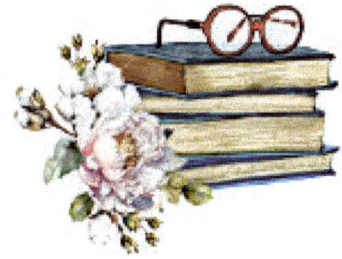

MIND: How did I do today, with treating myself with kindness? What worked? What felt good? How did I take care of myself?

_____
_____
_____
_____
_____
_____
_____
_____
_____
_____

BODY: How did I or how will I prepare my body for a restful sleep tonight?

_____
_____
_____
_____
_____
_____
_____
_____
_____
_____

SPIRIT: What signs did I receive from Spirit today? What words of affirmation, mantra, or prayer will I say to myself, to quiet my mind and help me ease into a restful sleep?

_____
_____
_____
_____
_____
_____
_____
_____
_____
_____

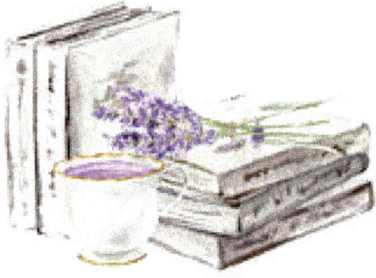

DAY NINE

✦

MORNING RITUAL

BODY: I will first take slow, deep breaths and do gentle stretches in bed. What other exercise or activity will I do? What nourishing foods will I provide myself with today?

_____
_____
_____
_____
_____
_____
_____
_____
_____

I am worthy of choosing relationships that are healthy

MIND: How will I choose to talk to myself and about myself today, even if something is off or not working? (I will practice self-acceptance and self-forgiveness, and be kind.)

_____
_____
_____
_____
_____
_____
_____
_____
_____

SPIRIT: I will be open to receiving signs from Spirit today. What inspirational affirmation, prayer, or mantra will guide me through my day?

_____
_____
_____
_____
_____
_____
_____
_____
_____
_____

23

DAY NINE

✦

EVENING RITUAL

MIND: How did I do today, with treating myself with kindness? What worked? What felt good? How did I take care of myself?

_____
_____
_____
_____
_____
_____
_____
_____
_____
_____

BODY: How did I or how will I prepare my body for a restful sleep tonight?

_____
_____
_____
_____
_____
_____
_____
_____
_____
_____

SPIRIT: What signs did I receive from Spirit today? What words of affirmation, mantra, or prayer will I say to myself, to quiet my mind and help me ease into a restful sleep?

_____
_____
_____
_____
_____
_____
_____
_____
_____
_____

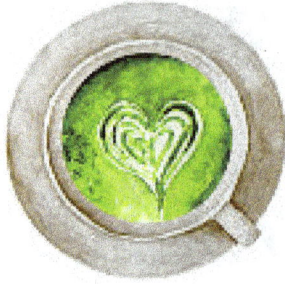

DAY TEN

✦

MORNING RITUAL

BODY: I will first take slow, deep breaths and do gentle stretches in bed. What other exercise or activity will I do? What nourishing foods will I provide myself with today?

_____
_____
_____
_____
_____
_____
_____
_____
_____

I will be gently supportive and encouraging with my Self

MIND: How will I choose to talk to myself and about myself today, even if something is off or not working? (I will practice self-acceptance and self-forgiveness, and be kind.)

_____
_____
_____
_____
_____
_____
_____
_____
_____
_____
_____

SPIRIT: I will be open to receiving signs from Spirit today. What inspirational affirmation, prayer, or mantra will guide me through my day?

_____
_____
_____
_____
_____
_____
_____
_____

DAY TEN

✦

EVENING RITUAL

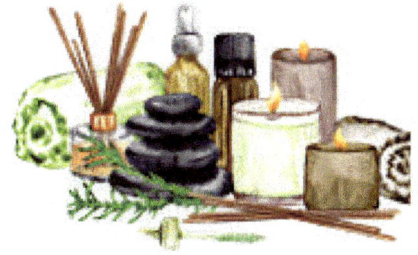

MIND: How did I do today, with treating myself with kindness? What worked? What felt good? How did I take care of myself?

_____
_____
_____
_____
_____
_____
_____
_____
_____
_____

BODY: How did I or how will I prepare my body for a restful sleep tonight?

_____
_____
_____
_____
_____
_____
_____
_____
_____
_____

SPIRIT: What signs did I receive from Spirit today? What words of affirmation, mantra, or prayer will I say to myself, to quiet my mind and help me ease into a restful sleep?

_____
_____
_____
_____
_____
_____
_____
_____
_____
_____

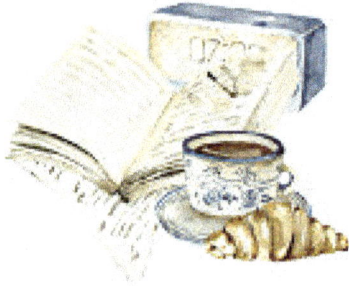

DAY ELEVEN

✦

MORNING RITUAL

BODY: I will first take slow, deep breaths and do gentle stretches in bed. What other exercise or activity will I do? What nourishing foods will I provide myself with today?

_____
_____
_____
_____
_____
_____
_____
_____
_____

I am the best person to decide what lifts my spirits

MIND: How will I choose to talk to myself and about myself today, even if something is off or not working? (I will practice self-acceptance and self-forgiveness, and be kind.)

_____
_____
_____
_____
_____
_____
_____
_____
_____

SPIRIT: I will be open to receiving signs from Spirit today. What inspirational affirmation, prayer, or mantra will guide me through my day?

_____
_____
_____
_____
_____
_____
_____
_____
_____

DAY ELEVEN

✦

EVENING RITUAL

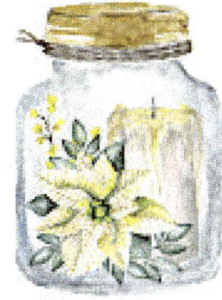

MIND: How did I do today, with treating myself with kindness? What worked? What felt good? How did I take care of myself?

_____
_____
_____
_____
_____
_____
_____
_____
_____
_____

BODY: How did I or how will I prepare my body for a restful sleep tonight?

_____
_____
_____
_____
_____
_____
_____
_____
_____
_____

SPIRIT: What signs did I receive from Spirit today? What words of affirmation, mantra, or prayer will I say to myself, to quiet my mind and help me ease into a restful sleep?

_____
_____
_____
_____
_____
_____
_____
_____
_____
_____

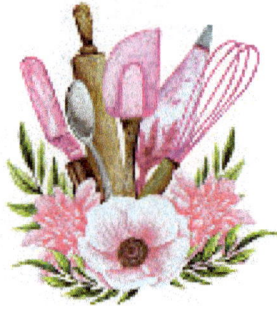

DAY TWELVE

✦

MORNING RITUAL

BODY: I will first take slow, deep breaths and do gentle stretches in bed. What other exercise or activity will I do? What nourishing foods will I provide myself with today?

_____
_____
_____
_____
_____
_____
_____
_____
_____

Your task is not to seek love, but merely to seek all the barriers within yourself that you have built against it

— Rumi

MIND: How will I choose to talk to myself and about myself today, even if something is off or not working? (I will practice self-acceptance and self-forgiveness, and be kind.)

_____
_____
_____
_____
_____
_____
_____
_____

SPIRIT: I will be open to receiving signs from Spirit today. What inspirational affirmation, prayer, or mantra will guide me through my day?

_____
_____
_____
_____
_____
_____
_____

DAY TWELVE

✦

EVENING RITUAL

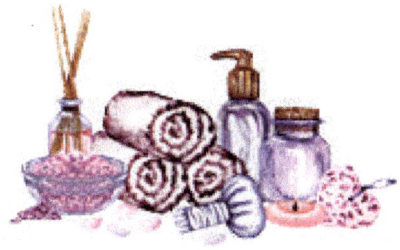

MIND: How did I do today, with treating myself with kindness? What worked? What felt good? How did I take care of myself?

_____
_____
_____
_____
_____
_____
_____
_____
_____

BODY: How did I or how will I prepare my body for a restful sleep tonight?

_____
_____
_____
_____
_____
_____
_____
_____
_____
_____

SPIRIT: What signs did I receive from Spirit today? What words of affirmation, mantra, or prayer will I say to myself, to quiet my mind and help me ease into a restful sleep?

_____
_____
_____
_____
_____
_____
_____
_____

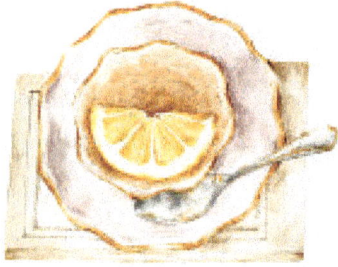

DAY THIRTEEN

✦

MORNING RITUAL

BODY: I will first take slow, deep breaths and do gentle stretches in bed. What other exercise or activity will I do? What nourishing foods will I provide myself with today?

_____
_____
_____
_____
_____
_____
_____
_____
_____

I choose to listen to my Higher Mind

MIND: How will I choose to talk to myself and about myself today, even if something is off or not working? (I will practice self-acceptance and self-forgiveness, and be kind.)

_____
_____
_____
_____
_____
_____
_____
_____

SPIRIT: I will be open to receiving signs from Spirit today. What inspirational affirmation, prayer, or mantra will guide me through my day?

_____
_____
_____
_____
_____
_____
_____
_____
_____

DAY THIRTEEN

✦

EVENING RITUAL

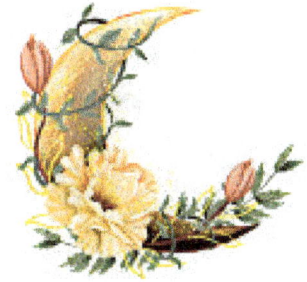

MIND: How did I do today, with treating myself with kindness? What worked? What felt good? How did I take care of myself?

_____
_____
_____
_____
_____
_____
_____
_____
_____

BODY: How did I or how will I prepare my body for a restful sleep tonight?

_____
_____
_____
_____
_____
_____
_____
_____
_____
_____
_____

SPIRIT: What signs did I receive from Spirit today? What words of affirmation, mantra, or prayer will I say to myself, to quiet my mind and help me ease into a restful sleep?

_____
_____
_____
_____
_____
_____
_____
_____
_____

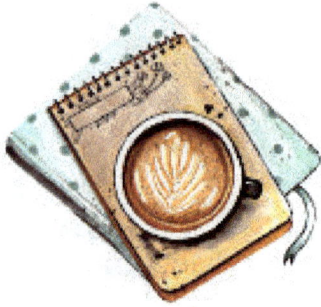

DAY FOURTEEN

✦

MORNING RITUAL

BODY: I will first take slow, deep breaths and do gentle stretches in bed. What other exercise or activity will I do? What nourishing foods will I provide myself with today?

_____
_____
_____
_____
_____
_____
_____
_____

What is it you plan to do with your one wild and precious life?

– Mary Oliver

MIND: How will I choose to talk to myself and about myself today, even if something is off or not working? (I will practice self-acceptance and self-forgiveness, and be kind.)

_____
_____
_____
_____
_____
_____
_____
_____

SPIRIT: I will be open to receiving signs from Spirit today. What inspirational affirmation, prayer, or mantra will guide me through my day?

_____
_____
_____
_____
_____
_____
_____
_____

DAY FOURTEEN

✦

EVENING RITUAL

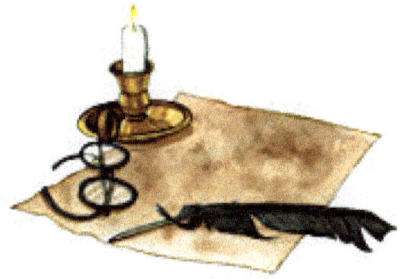

MIND: How did I do today, with treating myself with kindness? What worked? What felt good? How did I take care of myself?

_____
_____
_____
_____
_____
_____
_____
_____
_____

BODY: How did I or how will I prepare my body for a restful sleep tonight?

_____
_____
_____
_____
_____
_____
_____
_____
_____
_____
_____

SPIRIT: What signs did I receive from Spirit today? What words of affirmation, mantra, or prayer will I say to myself, to quiet my mind and help me ease into a restful sleep?

_____
_____
_____
_____
_____
_____
_____
_____
_____
_____

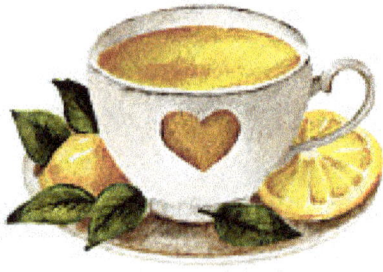

DAY FIFTEEN

✦

MORNING RITUAL

BODY: I will first take slow, deep breaths and do gentle stretches in bed. What other exercise or activity will I do? What nourishing foods will I provide myself with today?

_____
_____
_____
_____
_____
_____
_____
_____

I breathe in peace ~ I breathe out tension

MIND: How will I choose to talk to myself and about myself today, even if something is off or not working? (I will practice self-acceptance and self-forgiveness, and be kind.)

_____
_____
_____
_____
_____
_____
_____
_____

SPIRIT: I will be open to receiving signs from Spirit today. What inspirational affirmation, prayer, or mantra will guide me through my day?

_____
_____
_____
_____
_____
_____
_____
_____

DAY FIFTEEN

✦

EVENING RITUAL

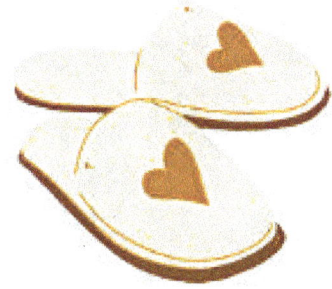

MIND: How did I do today, with treating myself with kindness? What worked? What felt good? How did I take care of myself?

_____
_____
_____
_____
_____
_____
_____
_____
_____

BODY: How did I or how will I prepare my body for a restful sleep tonight?

_____
_____
_____
_____
_____
_____
_____
_____
_____
_____
_____

SPIRIT: What signs did I receive from Spirit today? What words of affirmation, mantra, or prayer will I say to myself, to quiet my mind and help me ease into a restful sleep?

_____
_____
_____
_____
_____
_____
_____
_____

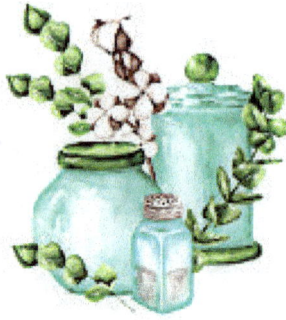

DAY SIXTEEN

✦

MORNING RITUAL

BODY: I will first take slow, deep breaths and do gentle stretches in bed. What other exercise or activity will I do? What nourishing foods will I provide myself with today?

_____
_____
_____
_____
_____
_____
_____
_____
_____

I breathe in self-compassion ~ I breathe out self-harm

MIND: How will I choose to talk to myself and about myself today, even if something is off or not working? (I will practice self-acceptance and self-forgiveness, and be kind.)

_____
_____
_____
_____
_____
_____
_____
_____
_____

SPIRIT: I will be open to receiving signs from Spirit today. What inspirational affirmation, prayer, or mantra will guide me through my day?

_____
_____
_____
_____
_____
_____
_____
_____

DAY SIXTEEN

✦

EVENING RITUAL

Sweet Dreams

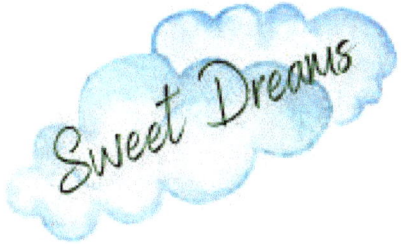

MIND: How did I do today, with treating myself with kindness? What worked? What felt good? How did I take care of myself?

_____
_____
_____
_____
_____
_____
_____
_____
_____
_____

BODY: How did I or how will I prepare my body for a restful sleep tonight?

_____
_____
_____
_____
_____
_____
_____
_____
_____
_____
_____

SPIRIT: What signs did I receive from Spirit today? What words of affirmation, mantra, or prayer will I say to myself, to quiet my mind and help me ease into a restful sleep?

_____
_____
_____
_____
_____
_____
_____
_____

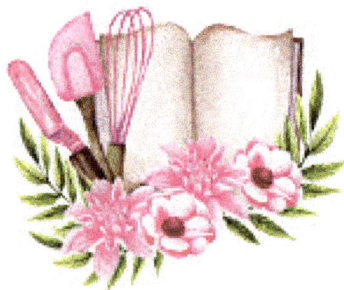

DAY SEVENTEEN

✦

MORNING RITUAL

BODY: I will first take slow, deep breaths and do gentle stretches in bed. What other exercise or activity will I do? What nourishing foods will I provide myself with today?

_____
_____
_____
_____
_____
_____
_____
_____

I breathe in love ~ I breathe out fear

MIND: How will I choose to talk to myself and about myself today, even if something is off or not working? (I will practice self-acceptance and self-forgiveness, and be kind.)

_____
_____
_____
_____
_____
_____
_____
_____

SPIRIT: I will be open to receiving signs from Spirit today. What inspirational affirmation, prayer, or mantra will guide me through my day?

_____
_____
_____
_____
_____
_____
_____
_____

DAY SEVENTEEN

✦

EVENING RITUAL

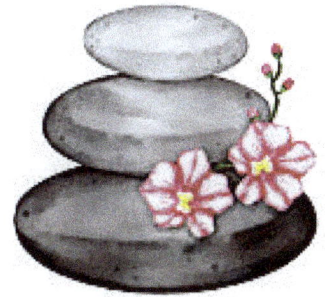

MIND: How did I do today, with treating myself with kindness? What worked? What felt good? How did I take care of myself?

_____
_____
_____
_____
_____
_____
_____
_____
_____
_____

BODY: How did I or how will I prepare my body for a restful sleep tonight?

_____
_____
_____
_____
_____
_____
_____
_____
_____
_____

SPIRIT: What signs did I receive from Spirit today? What words of affirmation, mantra, or prayer will I say to myself, to quiet my mind and help me ease into a restful sleep?

_____
_____
_____
_____
_____
_____
_____
_____
_____
_____

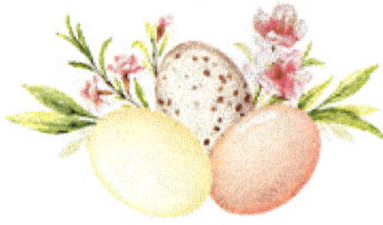

DAY EIGHTEEN

✦

MORNING RITUAL

BODY: I will first take slow, deep breaths and do gentle stretches in bed. What other exercise or activity will I do? What nourishing foods will I provide myself with today?

_____
_____
_____
_____
_____
_____
_____
_____

You will love again, the stranger who was yourself

– David Walcott

MIND: How will I choose to talk to myself and about myself today, even if something is off or not working? (I will practice self-acceptance and self-forgiveness, and be kind.)

_____
_____
_____
_____
_____
_____
_____

SPIRIT: I will be open to receiving signs from Spirit today. What inspirational affirmation, prayer, or mantra will guide me through my day?

_____
_____
_____
_____
_____
_____
_____
_____

DAY EIGHTEEN

✦

EVENING RITUAL

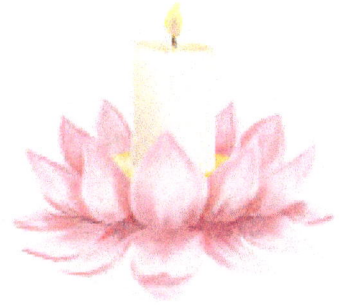

MIND: How did I do today, with treating myself with kindness? What worked? What felt good? How did I take care of myself?

_____
_____
_____
_____
_____
_____
_____
_____
_____
_____

BODY: How did I or how will I prepare my body for a restful sleep tonight?

_____
_____
_____
_____
_____
_____
_____
_____
_____
_____

SPIRIT: What signs did I receive from Spirit today? What words of affirmation, mantra, or prayer will I say to myself, to quiet my mind and help me ease into a restful sleep?

_____
_____
_____
_____
_____
_____
_____
_____

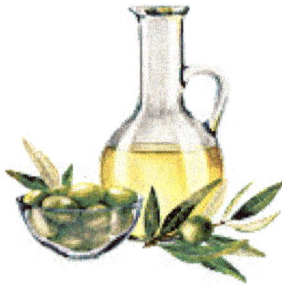

DAY NINETEEN

✦

MORNING RITUAL

BODY: I will first take slow, deep breaths and do gentle stretches in bed. What other exercise or activity will I do? What nourishing foods will I provide myself with today?

_____
_____
_____
_____
_____
_____
_____
_____

I will be present and observe ~ without comment or judgment

MIND: How will I choose to talk to myself and about myself today, even if something is off or not working? (I will practice self-acceptance and self-forgiveness, and be kind.)

_____
_____
_____
_____
_____
_____
_____
_____

SPIRIT: I will be open to receiving signs from Spirit today. What inspirational affirmation, prayer, or mantra will guide me through my day?

_____
_____
_____
_____
_____
_____
_____
_____
_____

DAY NINETEEN

✦

EVENING RITUAL

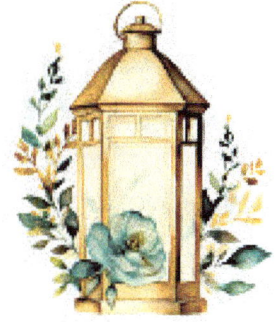

MIND: How did I do today, with treating myself with kindness? What worked? What felt good? How did I take care of myself?

_____
_____
_____
_____
_____
_____
_____
_____
_____

BODY: How did I or how will I prepare my body for a restful sleep tonight?

_____
_____
_____
_____
_____
_____
_____
_____
_____

SPIRIT: What signs did I receive from Spirit today? What words of affirmation, mantra, or prayer will I say to myself, to quiet my mind and help me ease into a restful sleep?

_____
_____
_____
_____
_____
_____
_____
_____
_____

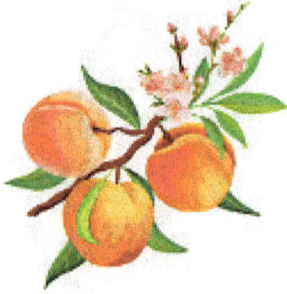

DAY TWENTY

✦

MORNING RITUAL

BODY: I will first take slow, deep breaths and do gentle stretches in bed. What other exercise or activity will I do? What nourishing foods will I provide myself with today?

_____
_____
_____
_____
_____
_____
_____
_____

Under any circumstance, simply do your best and you will avoid self-judgment, self-abuse, and regret

– Don Miguel Ruiz

MIND: How will I choose to talk to myself and about myself today, even if something is off or not working? (I will practice self-acceptance and self-forgiveness, and be kind.)

_____
_____
_____
_____
_____
_____
_____
_____

SPIRIT: I will be open to receiving signs from Spirit today. What inspirational affirmation, prayer, or mantra will guide me through my day?

_____
_____
_____
_____
_____
_____
_____
_____

DAY TWENTY

✦

EVENING RITUAL

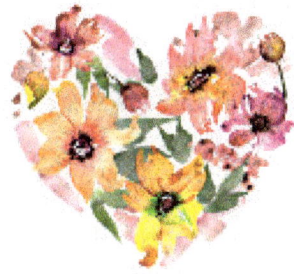

MIND: How did I do today, with treating myself with kindness? What worked? What felt good? How did I take care of myself?

_____
_____
_____
_____
_____
_____
_____
_____
_____

BODY: How did I or how will I prepare my body for a restful sleep tonight?

_____
_____
_____
_____
_____
_____
_____
_____
_____
_____

SPIRIT: What signs did I receive from Spirit today? What words of affirmation, mantra, or prayer will I say to myself, to quiet my mind and help me ease into a restful sleep?

_____
_____
_____
_____
_____
_____
_____
_____

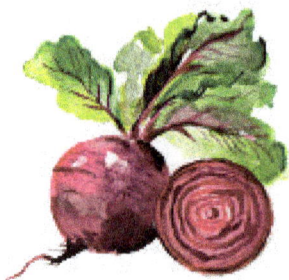

DAY TWENTY-ONE

✦

MORNING RITUAL

BODY: I will first take slow, deep breaths and do gentle stretches in bed. What other exercise or activity will I do? What nourishing foods will I provide myself with today?

_____
_____
_____
_____
_____
_____
_____
_____

I forgive all parts of my Self

MIND: How will I choose to talk to myself and about myself today, even if something is off or not working? (I will practice self-acceptance and self-forgiveness, and be kind.)

_____
_____
_____
_____
_____
_____
_____
_____

SPIRIT: I will be open to receiving signs from Spirit today. What inspirational affirmation, prayer, or mantra will guide me through my day?

_____
_____
_____
_____
_____
_____
_____

DAY TWENTY-ONE

✦

EVENING RITUAL

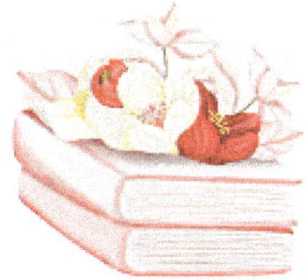

MIND: How did I do today, with treating myself with kindness? What worked? What felt good? How did I take care of myself?

_____
_____
_____
_____
_____
_____
_____
_____
_____
_____

BODY: How did I or how will I prepare my body for a restful sleep tonight?

_____
_____
_____
_____
_____
_____
_____
_____
_____

SPIRIT: What signs did I receive from Spirit today? What words of affirmation, mantra, or prayer will I say to myself, to quiet my mind and help me ease into a restful sleep?

_____
_____
_____
_____
_____
_____
_____
_____
_____
_____

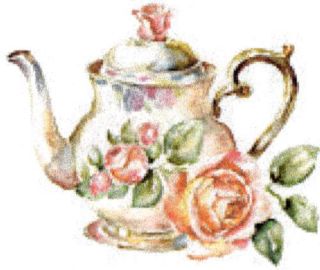

DAY TWENTY-TWO

✦

MORNING RITUAL

BODY: I will first take slow, deep breaths and do gentle stretches in bed. What other exercise or activity will I do? What nourishing foods will I provide myself with today?

_____
_____
_____
_____
_____
_____
_____
_____
_____

I choose to live my life with purpose and intention

MIND: How will I choose to talk to myself and about myself today, even if something is off or not working? (I will practice self-acceptance and self-forgiveness, and be kind.)

_____
_____
_____
_____
_____
_____
_____
_____
_____
_____

SPIRIT: I will be open to receiving signs from Spirit today. What inspirational affirmation, prayer, or mantra will guide me through my day?

_____
_____
_____
_____
_____
_____
_____
_____
_____
_____

DAY TWENTY-TWO

✦

EVENING RITUAL

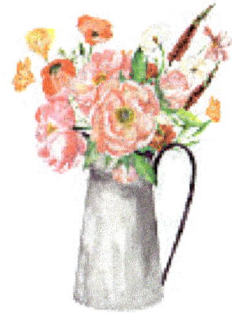

MIND: How did I do today, with treating myself with kindness? What worked? What felt good? How did I take care of myself?

_____
_____
_____
_____
_____
_____
_____
_____
_____

BODY: How did I or how will I prepare my body for a restful sleep tonight?

_____
_____
_____
_____
_____
_____
_____
_____
_____
_____
_____

SPIRIT: What signs did I receive from Spirit today? What words of affirmation, mantra, or prayer will I say to myself, to quiet my mind and help me ease into a restful sleep?

_____
_____
_____
_____
_____
_____
_____
_____

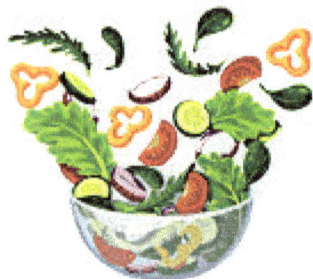

DAY TWENTY-THREE

✦

MORNING RITUAL

BODY: I will first take slow, deep breaths and do gentle stretches in bed. What other exercise or activity will I do? What nourishing foods will I provide myself with today?

_____
_____
_____
_____
_____
_____
_____
_____

Love yourself first and everything else falls into line

– Lucille Ball

MIND: How will I choose to talk to myself and about myself today, even if something is off or not working? (I will practice self-acceptance and self-forgiveness, and be kind.)

_____
_____
_____
_____
_____
_____
_____
_____

SPIRIT: I will be open to receiving signs from Spirit today. What inspirational affirmation, prayer, or mantra will guide me through my day?

_____
_____
_____
_____
_____
_____
_____
_____

DAY TWENTY-THREE

✦

EVENING RITUAL

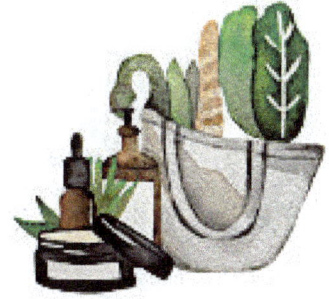

MIND: How did I do today, with treating myself with kindness? What worked? What felt good? How did I take care of myself?

_____
_____
_____
_____
_____
_____
_____
_____
_____

BODY: How did I or how will I prepare my body for a restful sleep tonight?

_____
_____
_____
_____
_____
_____
_____
_____
_____
_____
_____

SPIRIT: What signs did I receive from Spirit today? What words of affirmation, mantra, or prayer will I say to myself, to quiet my mind and help me ease into a restful sleep?

_____
_____
_____
_____
_____
_____
_____
_____

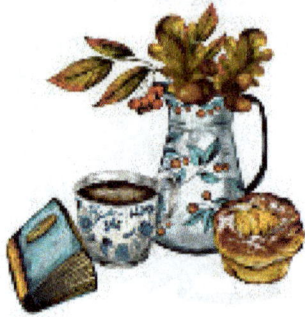

DAY TWENTY-FOUR

✦

MORNING RITUAL

BODY: I will first take slow, deep breaths and do gentle stretches in bed. What other exercise or activity will I do? What nourishing foods will I provide myself with today?

_____
_____
_____
_____
_____
_____
_____
_____

I choose to love my Self

MIND: How will I choose to talk to myself and about myself today, even if something is off or not working? (I will practice self-acceptance and self-forgiveness, and be kind.)

_____
_____
_____
_____
_____
_____
_____
_____

SPIRIT: I will be open to receiving signs from Spirit today. What inspirational affirmation, prayer, or mantra will guide me through my day?

_____
_____
_____
_____
_____
_____
_____
_____
_____
_____

53

DAY TWENTY-FOUR

✦

EVENING RITUAL

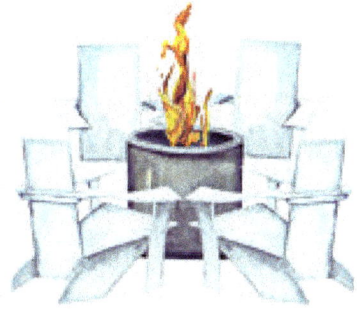

MIND: How did I do today, with treating myself with kindness? What worked? What felt good? How did I take care of myself?

_____
_____
_____
_____
_____
_____
_____
_____

BODY: How did I or how will I prepare my body for a restful sleep tonight?

_____
_____
_____
_____
_____
_____
_____
_____
_____

SPIRIT: What signs did I receive from Spirit today? What words of affirmation, mantra, or prayer will I say to myself, to quiet my mind and help me ease into a restful sleep?

_____
_____
_____
_____
_____
_____
_____
_____

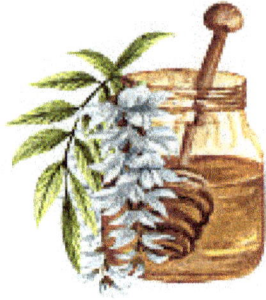

DAY TWENTY-FIVE

✦

MORNING RITUAL

BODY: I will first take slow, deep breaths and do gentle stretches in bed. What other exercise or activity will I do? What nourishing foods will I provide myself with today?

_____
_____
_____
_____
_____
_____
_____
_____

I am fully present in this precious moment of life

MIND: How will I choose to talk to myself and about myself today, even if something is off or not working? (I will practice self-acceptance and self-forgiveness, and be kind.)

_____
_____
_____
_____
_____
_____
_____
_____

SPIRIT: I will be open to receiving signs from Spirit today. What inspirational affirmation, prayer, or mantra will guide me through my day?

_____
_____
_____
_____
_____
_____
_____
_____

DAY TWENTY-FIVE

✦

EVENING RITUAL

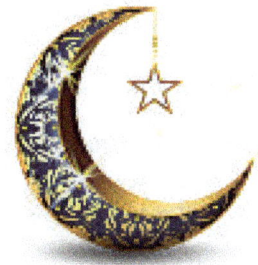

MIND: How did I do today, with treating myself with kindness? What worked? What felt good? How did I take care of myself?

_____
_____
_____
_____
_____
_____
_____
_____
_____

BODY: How did I or how will I prepare my body for a restful sleep tonight?

_____
_____
_____
_____
_____
_____
_____
_____
_____
_____

SPIRIT: What signs did I receive from Spirit today? What words of affirmation, mantra, or prayer will I say to myself, to quiet my mind and help me ease into a restful sleep?

_____
_____
_____
_____
_____
_____
_____

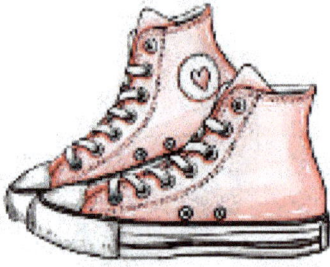

DAY TWENTY-SIX

✦

MORNING RITUAL

BODY: I will first take slow, deep breaths and do gentle stretches in bed. What other exercise or activity will I do? What nourishing foods will I provide myself with today?

_____
_____
_____
_____
_____
_____
_____
_____

I am my own best advocate for living a healthy life

MIND: How will I choose to talk to myself and about myself today, even if something is off or not working? (I will practice self-acceptance and self-forgiveness, and be kind.)

_____
_____
_____
_____
_____
_____
_____
_____

SPIRIT: I will be open to receiving signs from Spirit today. What inspirational affirmation, prayer, or mantra will guide me through my day?

_____
_____
_____
_____
_____
_____
_____
_____
_____

DAY TWENTY-SIX

✦

EVENING RITUAL

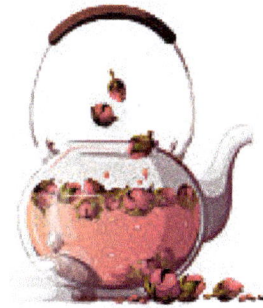

MIND: How did I do today, with treating myself with kindness? What worked? What felt good? How did I take care of myself?

_____
_____
_____
_____
_____
_____
_____
_____

BODY: How did I or how will I prepare my body for a restful sleep tonight?

_____
_____
_____
_____
_____
_____
_____
_____
_____

SPIRIT: What signs did I receive from Spirit today? What words of affirmation, mantra, or prayer will I say to myself, to quiet my mind and help me ease into a restful sleep?

_____
_____
_____
_____
_____
_____
_____
_____

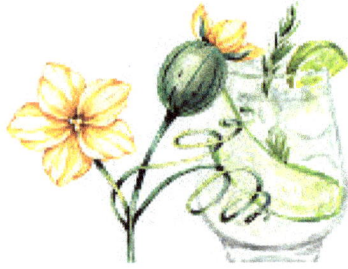

DAY TWENTY-SEVEN

✦

MORNING RITUAL

BODY: I will first take slow, deep breaths and do gentle stretches in bed. What other exercise or activity will I do? What nourishing foods will I provide myself with today?

_____
_____
_____
_____
_____
_____
_____
_____

I choose to speak about myself and others with loving kindness

MIND: How will I choose to talk to myself and about myself today, even if something is off or not working? (I will practice self-acceptance and self-forgiveness, and be kind.)

_____
_____
_____
_____
_____
_____
_____
_____

SPIRIT: I will be open to receiving signs from Spirit today. What inspirational affirmation, prayer, or mantra will guide me through my day?

_____
_____
_____
_____
_____
_____
_____
_____

DAY TWENTY-SEVEN

✦

EVENING RITUAL

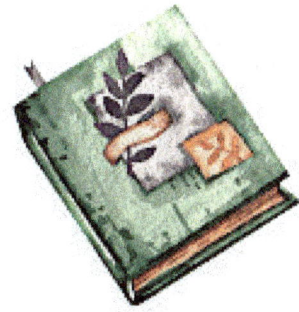

MIND: How did I do today, with treating myself with kindness? What worked? What felt good? How did I take care of myself?

_____
_____
_____
_____
_____
_____
_____
_____
_____

BODY: How did I or how will I prepare my body for a restful sleep tonight?

_____
_____
_____
_____
_____
_____
_____
_____
_____
_____

SPIRIT: What signs did I receive from Spirit today? What words of affirmation, mantra, or prayer will I say to myself, to quiet my mind and help me ease into a restful sleep?

_____
_____
_____
_____
_____
_____
_____
_____

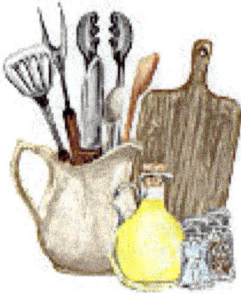

DAY TWENTY-EIGHT

✦

MORNING RITUAL

BODY: I will first take slow, deep breaths and do gentle stretches in bed. What other exercise or activity will I do? What nourishing foods will I provide myself with today?

_____
_____
_____
_____
_____
_____
_____
_____
_____

I celebrate my unique expression of Self

MIND: How will I choose to talk to myself and about myself today, even if something is off or not working? (I will practice self-acceptance and self-forgiveness, and be kind.)

_____
_____
_____
_____
_____
_____
_____
_____
_____

SPIRIT: I will be open to receiving signs from Spirit today. What inspirational affirmation, prayer, or mantra will guide me through my day?

_____
_____
_____
_____
_____
_____
_____
_____
_____

DAY TWENTY-EIGHT

✦

EVENING RITUAL

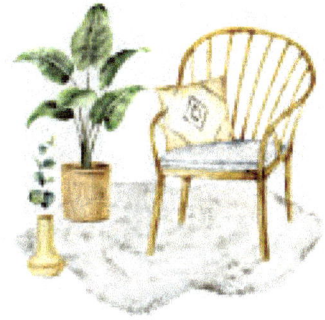

MIND: How did I do today, with treating myself with kindness? What worked? What felt good? How did I take care of myself?

_____
_____
_____
_____
_____
_____
_____
_____
_____

BODY: How did I or how will I prepare my body for a restful sleep tonight?

_____
_____
_____
_____
_____
_____
_____
_____
_____
_____

SPIRIT: What signs did I receive from Spirit today? What words of affirmation, mantra, or prayer will I say to myself, to quiet my mind and help me ease into a restful sleep?

_____
_____
_____
_____
_____
_____
_____
_____

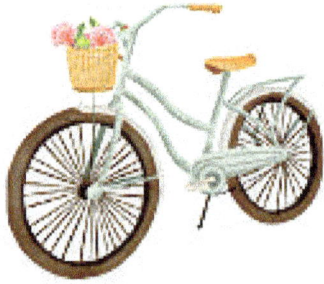

DAY TWENTY-NINE

✦

MORNING RITUAL

BODY: I will first take slow, deep breaths and do gentle stretches in bed. What other exercise or activity will I do? What nourishing foods will I provide myself with today?

_____
_____
_____
_____
_____
_____
_____
_____

This being human is a guest house ~ every morning a new arrival

– Rumi

MIND: How will I choose to talk to myself and about myself today, even if something is off or not working? (I will practice self-acceptance and self-forgiveness, and be kind.)

_____
_____
_____
_____
_____
_____
_____
_____

SPIRIT: I will be open to receiving signs from Spirit today. What inspirational affirmation, prayer, or mantra will guide me through my day?

_____
_____
_____
_____
_____
_____
_____

DAY TWENTY-NINE
✦
EVENING RITUAL

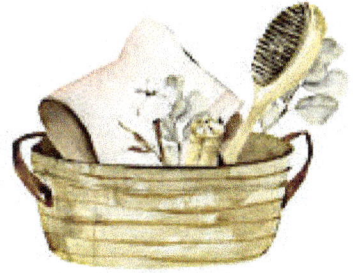

MIND: How did I do today, with treating myself with kindness? What worked? What felt good? How did I take care of myself?

_____
_____
_____
_____
_____
_____
_____
_____
_____
_____

BODY: How did I or how will I prepare my body for a restful sleep tonight?

_____
_____
_____
_____
_____
_____
_____
_____
_____
_____

SPIRIT: What signs did I receive from Spirit today? What words of affirmation, mantra, or prayer will I say to myself, to quiet my mind and help me ease into a restful sleep?

_____
_____
_____
_____
_____
_____
_____

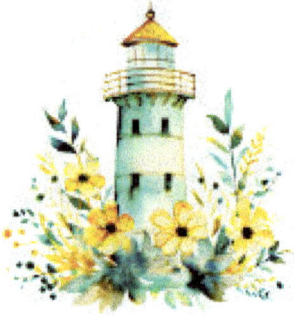

DAY THIRTY

✦

MORNING RITUAL

BODY: I will first take slow, deep breaths and do gentle stretches in bed. What other exercise or activity will I do? What nourishing foods will I provide myself with today?

_____
_____
_____
_____
_____
_____
_____
_____

I am the lighthouse ~ I shine from within

MIND: How will I choose to talk to myself and about myself today, even if something is off or not working? (I will practice self-acceptance and self-forgiveness, and be kind.)

_____
_____
_____
_____
_____
_____
_____
_____

SPIRIT: I will be open to receiving signs from Spirit today. What inspirational affirmation, prayer, or mantra will guide me through my day?

_____
_____
_____
_____
_____
_____
_____
_____

DAY THIRTY

✦

EVENING RITUAL

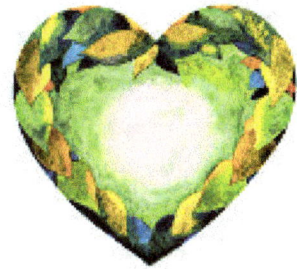

MIND: How did I do today, with treating myself with kindness? What worked? What felt good? How did I take care of myself?

_____
_____
_____
_____
_____
_____
_____
_____
_____
_____

BODY: How did I or how will I prepare my body for a restful sleep tonight?

_____
_____
_____
_____
_____
_____
_____
_____
_____
_____

SPIRIT: What signs did I receive from Spirit today? What words of affirmation, mantra, or prayer will I say to myself, to quiet my mind and help me ease into a restful sleep?

_____
_____
_____
_____
_____
_____
_____
_____

JOURNAL

JOURNAL

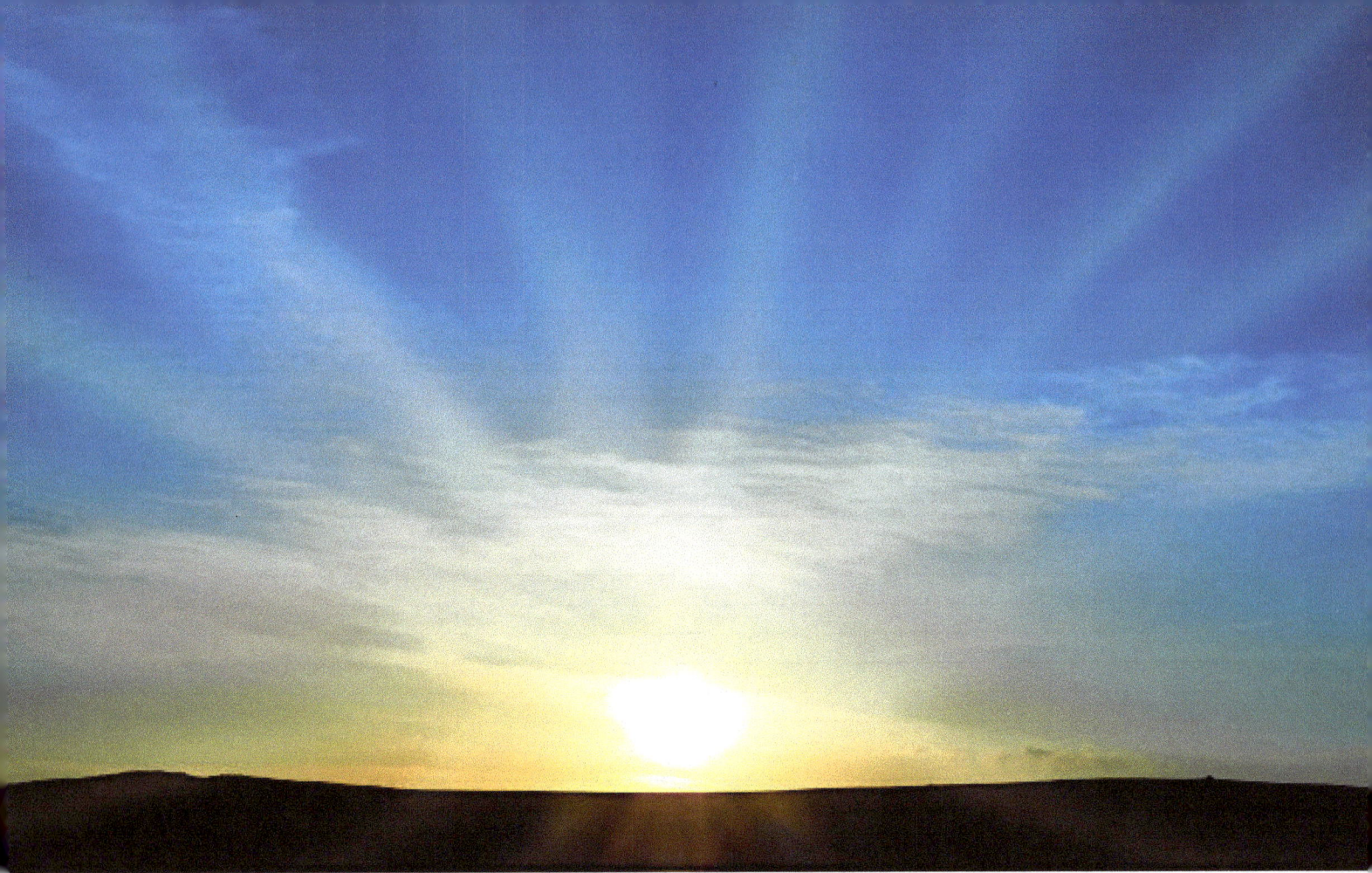

CONGRATULATIONS!

You did it! You took the time to fully commit to your Self and invest in becoming your own best advocate for healthy living. Celebrate *you*!

Now, let's grow the self-care circle. In the spirit of "paying it forward," if doing this Bookending Your Day practice worked for you in any way, think of sharing it with those you think might benefit as well.

Just as the only day we really have is today, the only locus of control we have in life is how we care for ourselves and others. This is what we can do; we can be as loving of ourselves as we would be with our loved ones. How we treat ourselves has a ripple effect. When we practice self-care, everyone benefits -- our family, our friends, our co-workers. We are all in this together, this experience called *Life*! Shine and radiate from within, and outward to encompass your inner circle and beyond, to the whole world!

Be the lighthouse and let your light fully shine!

Faith Burrington Jones

Fear of confrontation used to silence me.
Self love raised my voice.

Fear of failure used to immobilize me.
Self love emboldened me.

Fear of judgment used to consume me.
Self love made me whole.

Fear of abandonment used to anchor me.
Self love helped me set sail.

– Melody Godfred

Self Love Poetry: For Thinkers & Feelers

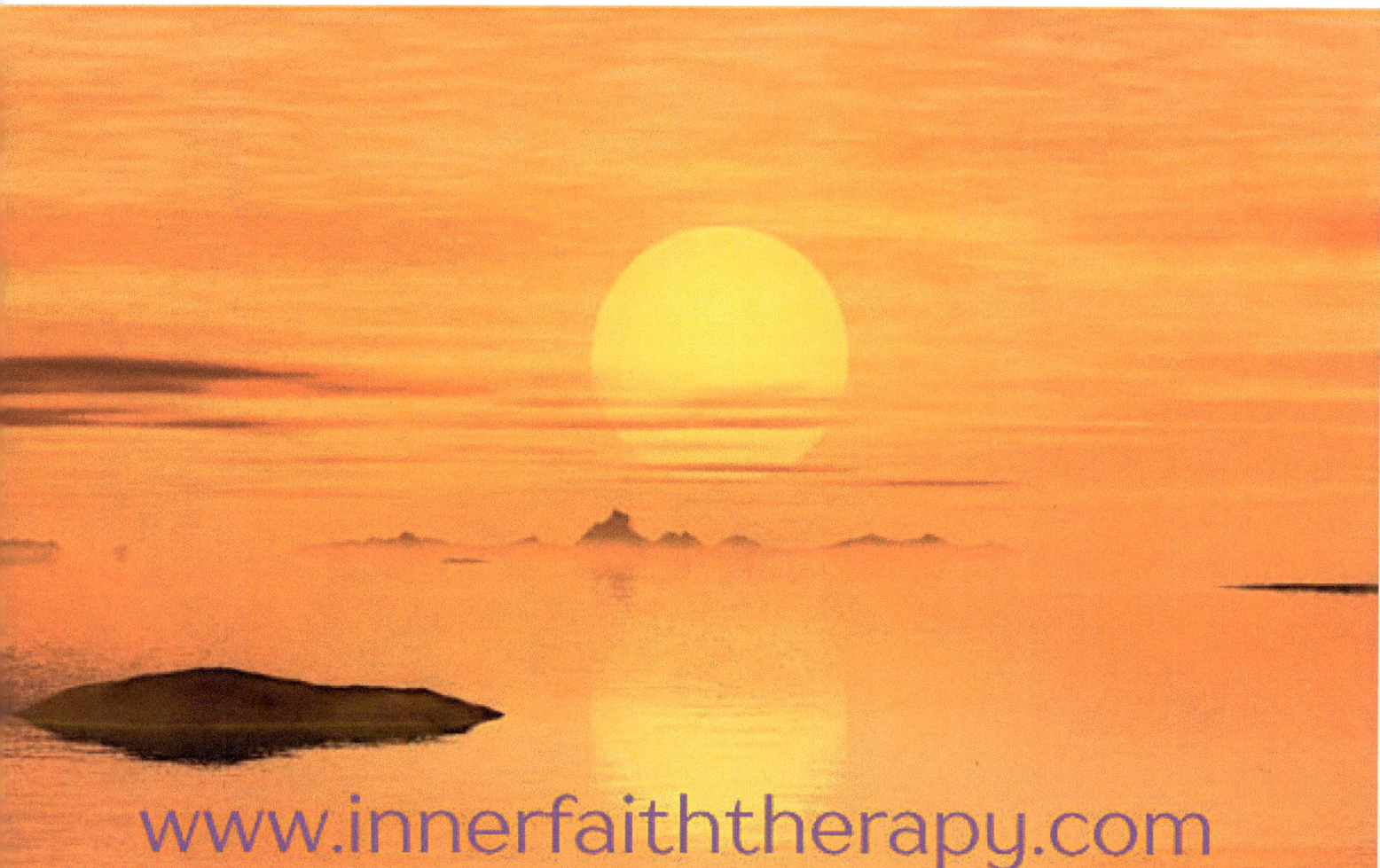

www.innerfaiththerapy.com

www.ingramcontent.com/pod-product-compliance
Lightning Source LLC
Chambersburg PA
CBHW052117020426

42335CB00021B/2810